Just the 50 Tips & Ideas

to longer, healthier hair

The Lush Long Hair Care Guide

Just the 50 Tips & Ideas to longer, healthier hair

The Lush Long Hair Care Guide

Allison Tyson

Copyright © 2012 Allison Tyson

Limited Edition

www.thelushlonghaircareguide.com

Before you start your journey to longer luscious hair, take a photo* of your hair.

Place photo of your hair here

*Back of the head shots are best

Hair Journey Start Date:

Goal Length:

Describe your hair:

Disclaimer

All material within this publication is for information purposes only.

This book is not intended to be a substitute for taking proper medical advice and should not be relied upon in this way. The author cannot accept any responsibility for illness arising from the failure to seek professional medical advice.

The information contained herein is not intended to cover all possible uses, directions, precautions, warnings, drug interactions, allergic reactions or adverse effects. If you have questions about the recommendations suggested, please seek the professional advice from your doctor, pharmacist or health provider before commencing any treatments.

Table of Contents

Introduction

Let me start by saying, I have had my share of bad hair experiences. I wrote my first book *The Lush Long Hair Care Guide* after years of searching for answers and having horrible hair. I could not stand looking at my hair in the mirror or let alone have anyone touch it. I needed to do something about it and I needed to do it NOW!

Just the 50 Tips & Ideas is the book I originally planned to write. Fortunately, whilst writing it I realised that many of the answers I found, such as "eat Brazil nuts, they'll make your hair grow" or "take Biotin supplements they will stop your hair from being brittle" etc, did not delve into the *why* they work. I wanted to find the answers (or misinformation) behind all these claims made by friends, wives tales, folk lore and most of all the outrageous ones I was hearing about in the media and written on the bottle of the latest new beaut product that had just hit the shelves.

If you are looking for the answers <u>and</u> the *why* behind them, you are reading the wrong book. *Just the 50 Tips & Ideas* has only the summary answers of each chapter of *The Lush Long Hair Care Guide*, fifty tips and ideas that will help you improve the health of your hair, but it won't give you the long winded *why* to back them up. Think of it more as the hit 'single' released from a hot new album. *Just the 50 Tips & Ideas* is a small taste of *The Lush Long Hair Care Guide* but without all the facts to back up the answers to the *why*.

I have released *Just the 50 Tips & Ideas* as a <u>Limited Edition</u> booklet in the hope more people will be curious enough to want to know the *whys*, and because it's an easy to read and affordable alternative. But for a short time only.

Author's note: Hair is only hair

Hair is only hair, and for most of us it will grow back even after we continue to damage and torture it.

For some of us, our hair defines us and it can be emotionally devastating when our hair falls out or just looks and feels wrong. If you are at your wits end and threatening to shave it all off and start again, please try some or all of the tips and ideas listed before doing anything too drastic.

To achieve the longest, healthiest hair possible, you need to consider doing the following:

Stop hair breakage/damage before it happens

Minimising hair breakage will allow your hair to reach its maximum length. Protect your hair using specific types of products (as suggested in this book), as part of a hair care regime which can help reduce breakage and increase your hair length.

Increase the growth phase and lessen shedding

Using hair vitamins and mineral supplements to complement a healthy eating plan will naturally lengthen your hair's anagen phase and allow your hair to grow much longer before it enters the resting and shedding phases. Get plenty of rest and practise positive stress management.

Improve the health of your hair before it starts to grow

A healthy, bacteria-free, well-nourished scalp enables you to grow lush, long, healthy hair.

Best of luck, happy growing!!

Over 50 Tips and Ideas

Tip 1: Coconut oil can be used as the perfect daily moisturiser. Simply put a small amount in the palms of your hands, rub together and apply to hair strands to keep hair moisturised.

Tip 2: Experiment with different oils like olive, mineral, avocado, almond and jojoba to trial which ones are right for you and work best with your hair type.

Tip 3: Castor Oil has been used for centuries in India to assist hair growth and to thicken hair.

Idea 1: **Castor oil growth recipe**

Castor oil is quite thick and sticky so it needs to be blended with other oils to ensure it does not accidentally rip your hairs out whilst you massage with it.

1. Mix 50mls of Castor oil with 50mls of your favourite carrier oil (Coconut, Avocado, Almond, Jojoba or Olive oil).

2. Apply to your hair roots, massage into scalp and then leave on overnight (or for at least half an hour).

3. Shampoo hair to remove Castor Oil residue

4. For maximum effect use three times a week

Tip 4: Argan oil locks in moisture and cures hair of brittleness.

Tip 5: Any process which uses chemicals to alter the structure of the hair will compromise the internal structure of your hair, weakening it and making it more susceptible to further damage. Over time and with repeated use it will leave your hair dry, dull, weak or frizzy and at greater risk of damage from the daily hair care routine.

Tip 6: Using henna helps smooth the cuticle and your hair is naturally plumped with volume from within, taking on a thicker, stronger texture. Henna stains hair to the desired colour without chemically damaging the hair structure. It can leave hair feeling gritty so use a deep conditioning agent for a few days after application.

Idea 2: **Changing the shades of Henna**

Red Henna (Lawsonia inermis): Provides a red stain, deepen by mixing and letting sit overnight in an iron pot, or accent with burgundy streaks by adding raw beetroot juice. Copper piping or pennies will add brown hues to red Henna. Adding natural yoghurt to your henna mix will help make application easier and give you a creamier consistency.

Black Henna (Indigofera tinctoria): Gives a deep black colouring.

Hendigo: A mix of henna and indigo in varying quantities will give different shades of browns including chestnut and mahogany.

Neutral Henna (Cassia obovata): has a golden dye molecule that will stain dull blonde and gray hair yellow. Cassia treatments can be used on dark tresses for shine enhancement.

Tip 7: Bleaching the hair is a very harsh process and should be avoided. It compromises the internal hair structure and can have devastating results if you aren't careful. The lighter you take your hair from its natural colour, the more damage will occur. Natural alternatives to chemical bleaching include Cinnamon essential oil, Baking Soda, Honey, Sunshine and Lemon Citrus essential oil.

Idea 3: **Coconut oil presoak**

Presoaking your hair with coconut oil will help your hair survive the damage harsh bleach can have on your hair. Ultimately you will have less of the damage usually associated with having hair chemically lightened.

1. Two days before having your hair bleached or highlighted, oil your hair with coconut oil.

2. Apply a liberal amount of virgin coconut oil to your entire hair shaft, root to tip. Leave in and do not wash out.

3. There's no need to wash it out each night or morning until the day you are due to start the bleaching

4. It is optional whether or not to remove the oil before bleaching agents are applied to your hair. The oil should not effect the strength of the chemicals.

Tip 8: Regardless of whether you visit a hair salon or colour, bleach or perm your hair at home, chemical processing damages your hair.

Tip 9: Excessive friction from manual hairstyling, like over-zealous brushing, backcombing or teasing, can damage and affect the health of your hair. If you choose to brush your hair, do it gently. To test if your brush or technique is costing you precious hairs, brush dry hair over a white sink and check for breakage. For people with thinning hair, every hair counts, harsh brushing can often pull out hair that would not have come out had you not brushed it.

Tip 10: Raking the wrong type of brush through your hair and brushing when wet makes your hair highly vulnerable to damage. The best way to detangle hair following a wash is by using a wide-toothed comb. Try to avoid using a hair brush until your hair is almost dry. If you must brush, lubricate your hair first with your favourite oils.

Tip 11: Using your hands and a small amount of your favourite oil or conditioner to gently untangle knots is a lot gentler and less aggressive way to avoid pulling hairs out by the roots or snapping hair. Fingercombing in the shower will also enhance curls.

Tip 12: Feel a comb or brush bristles for any rough or sharp areas before you purchase it. Sharp seams and plastic nibs catch on delicate long hair and promote breakage. Buy handmade wood or seamless plastic combs which will glide through your hair without catching on fragile strands. A good way to check if your current comb or brush is damaging your hair is to stand over a white sink whilst you groom your hair, if there is a large number of hairs breaking off you'll see them.

Tip 13: Hair is like string and will start to unravel regardless of where you cut it. Try 1/2 cm trims (only when you need to) to maintain healthy ends. Clean ends tangle less and will break less. Your faster growing hairs will be trimmed back regularly so that slower growing hairs can 'catch up', giving you less wispy ends and a thicker hemline.

Tip 14: Find a hairdresser that knows how to micro-trim. Speak up when in the hairdresser's chair, your hairdresser will appreciate your input and you are less likely to leave with your hair butchered into a style you really did not want.

Tip 15: Use warm water to wash or clarify, this opens up your hair cuticles and helps your conditioner or herbal rinse to penetrate the hair. Use cool water on low pressure to rinse and to close the cuticle. Alternating between hot and cold whilst in the shower also improves circulation to the scalp.

Tip 16: Keep your body and hair hydrated by drinking plenty of fresh clean water. Monitor your water intake.

Tip 17: There are several water contaminants that can cause hair loss, if these contaminants are in your water, try using a filtered showerhead.

Tip 18: Protect hair with a swim cap when swimming in chlorine or salt water, saturate with water and oil before getting in the water and rinse with club soda afterwards. Wetting the hair with non-chlorinated water prior to swimming in pools and the ocean will lessen the amount of chlorine and salt water elements absorbed into the hair shaft.

Idea 4: **Baking Soda Shampoo Recipe**

An effective alternative to using Chelating shampoos to remove chlorine and mineral deposits from your hair

1. Mix 1/2 teaspoon baking soda in 1litre of water and pour onto your scalp

2. Gently massage baking soda rinse into your hair

3. Rinse hair with warm water

4. Condition hair and rinse again with Apple Cider Vinegar rinse.

Tip 19: Although not the most attractive accessory, swimming caps are well-suited for protecting hair. For those with long hair, caps can also help hair from dragging along during laps becoming prone to more tangles.

Tip 20: Some of us have hair that can be damaged by chemicals in shampoos. Alternatives to using your current shampoo regime are worth considering; you just need to find what works for you.

Idea 5: **Shampooing Alternatives**

•Shampoo bars or baby shampoos which are ph balanced.

•Organic shampoos, but check the ingredients first for hidden nasties.

•Baking Soda in place of shampoo will cleanse the hair just as effectively without stripping it of moisture, but may lighten hair.

•Pre-oiling the scalp and hair with your favorite oils prior to washing to prevent the protein loss in response to shampooing

•Adding Coconut oil to shampoo to lessen the harshness of your current shampoo.

•Experiment with conditioning your hair first then washing followed by more conditioner

•Only wash with a conditioner

•Shampooing less frequently may help avoiding drying hair out.

Tip 21: You can still have your crowning glory shine and glow without the use of alcohol based styling products. There are many natural alcohol-free gels and sprays out there. A light oiling with Argan or your favourite oil can keep hair from being flyaway. On its own or diluted with water into a spray bottle Aloe Vera works wonders as a natural styling agent.

Tip 22: Naturally healthy hair needs a natural approach. Look for cone free and sulfate free shampoos and conditioners that do not contain harsh chemicals. Alternatively, go natural and use an apple cider vinegar rinse to remove build up, baking soda shampoos and oils for frizz free hair and leave in conditioning.

Tip 23: Protein treatments put protein back into your hair but should always be followed with a deep conditioning treatment. Homemade Egg, Soy Sauce or Gelatin protein treatments will save you money and give good results.

Idea 6: **Raw Egg Protein Treatment Recipe**

Recommended once a month if your hair is not dry and brittle.

1.Separate the yolk from the whites of two eggs and beat.

Only use the yolk of the egg for your protein masque, the whites will cause excessive dryness.

2.Apply the yolk mixture to dry hair and leave on for 30mins

3.Gently rinse hair with warm water.

4.Always follow your protein treatment with a deep conditioning treatment

Tip 24: Unrefined Shea Butter is full of vitamins and is a natural moisturiser. Its emollient properties relieve scalp dryness and leaves hair feeling silky and soft.

Idea 7: **Deep Conditioning Recipe**

Shea Butter deep conditioning masque

Recommended once a fortnight if your hair is dry and brittle.

1.Blend 2 tablespoons of Shea Butter with 1 tbls Coconut oil, Avocado or Olive Oil and 1 tbls of your favourite All Natural conditioner.

2.Apply to damp hair and leave on for 1-4hrs.

3.Rinse hair. Shampoo and condition

Tip 25: Apple Cider Vinegar is an excellent clarifying rinse to remove build up and cleanse your scalp.

Idea 8: **ACV Rinse Recipe**

Use once a week after washing to clarify and remove build up

1.Combine one to two tablespoons of ACV with one cup of water.

2.After washing pour the rinse over your hair

3.Do not rinse out, the vinegar 'smell' will abate once your hair has dried

Caution: Never mix Apple Cider Vinegar with Baking powder you could 'melt' your hair!

Tip 26: Torturing hair into submission damages your hair and causes breakage. Trying to attain a style that may not suit you is time consuming, expensive and could be costing you precious hairs. It may be time to stop fighting genetics and accept your hair type. Embrace your curls, kinks or individual style.

Tip 27: Chemical relaxing or straightening is never to the benefit to your hair's health. Regardless of which method of straightening you use, this type of hairstyling is extremely damaging.

Tip 28: Using heat to style hair can cause damage and dry out hair. Use the cooler settings on your hairdryer or avoid heat styling altogether.

Tip 29: Showers that are too hot can damage your hair, keep showers and bath water warm, not hot.

Tip 30: Heat can aid deep conditioners to penetrate the hair shaft by opening the cuticle, being especially beneficial for conditioning treatments on dry hair.

Idea 9: **Coconut Oil Heat Treatment**

1.Apply warm Coconut Oil to scalp and damp hair

2.Heat a towel in the microwave for 1minute or until warm

3.Wrap hair in warm towel

The hot towel will open the cuticles and allow the Coconut Oil to penetrate deep inside the hair shaft

4.Leave on for 30mins then rinse, wash out or use as leave in conditioner

Tip 31: Sock buns give curls and volume to straight or limp hair without the use of damaging heat.

Idea 10: **How to make Sock Bun**

1.Cut the foot off a long sock and roll it into a donut shape.

2.Comb your hair into a not-too-tight ponytail on top of your head (either use a band you do not mind snipping off or wrap a finger-width strand of hair around your tail and pin into place).

3.Lightly moisturise the ponytail using your favourite oil

4.Put the end of your ponytail into the donut opening.

5.Tuck the end of your tail up into the outside of the sock donut.

6.Now roll the donut down your ponytail until it's flush against your scalp.

Try and spread the hair evenly over the donut ensuring it doesn't show through

7.You may want to secure the sock in place with a bobby pin.

8.Leave in for a couple of hours or overnight to set.

9.Remove the sock and reveal your luscious lovely sock-bun curls

Tip 32: A Doobie will protect your hair while you sleep, exercise or even whilst doing your chores! When you take the Doobie out you'll notice your hair feels smooth, straight and tangle-free.

Idea 11: **How to Doobie Your Hair**

1.Start with clean, air dried and combed hair.

2.Be sure to comb your hair all in the same direction (i.e., to one side)

3.Take the ends of your hair and 'wrap' around your head, as far as you can

(Longer hair may wrap around all the way or more than once).

4.Secure your hair with bobby pins to keep it in place.

5.Protect with a headband or bandanna.

Tip 33: Switch up your hair part lines alternating from side parts and centre parts. Find your new part and pin it down with bobby pins as soon as you get out of the shower (so that it dries parted to the side). This technique trains your hair to lay which ever way you want it to.

Tip 34: Loose braids and bunning your hair without the use of over tight elastic bands will save your hair from accidental breakage during the day. Mix up styles to avoid Hair Repetitive Stress Injuries (RSI), even placing your ponytail in different locations (high, low and to the side) helps.

Tip 35: Seek the expertise of your Health Practitioner to determine any vitamin and mineral deficiencies. In combination with a healthy eating plan it is critical you are getting the correct doses of the vitamins and minerals you need. Pregnant and Breastfeeding mums and children will require different recommended daily amounts.

Tip 36: Studies show a direct correlation to hair loss and vitamin D deficiency. Spending a few minutes in the Sun is enough to get your daily dose. Wear a hat to protect your hair (and face) from Sun exposure.

Tip 37: The nutritional benefits of nuts can't be overlooked, eat a variety of nuts for best hair growth. The fats they contain are healthy fats and they make a great snack idea.

Tip 38: Diet and hair are linked. Follow the healthy hair diet if you want healthy beautiful hair eat healthy foods, avoid crash diets, and eat adequate amounts of protein, carbohydrates, fruit and vegetables, low-fat dairy and 'good' fats for your body type or lifestyle. A dietician or your Health Provider can assist you in creating a hair healthy eating plan suitable to your individual needs.

Idea 12: **Conditioning Banana Hair Masque Recipe**

1.Freeze a banana; this makes it easier to mush.

2.Use a blender or food processor to puree the banana until it is liquefied (Make sure it's totally smooth otherwise you'll end up with banana chunks stuck in your hair).

3.Blend the banana with a mashed avocado and a teaspoon of Olive oil or Coconut Oil.

(Avocados are packed with fatty acids that will soften the hair)

4.Once blended, scoop the mixture on to your damp hair.

5.Cover with a shower cap or plastic wrap and relax for 15 minutes.

6.Rinse with cool water.

Tip 39: For the internal benefits of Molasses take 1 tablespoon of blackstrap molasses first thing in the morning. Be careful, some people find molasses can have a laxative effect.

Idea 13: **Topically applied Molasses hair rinse**

1.Add one tablespoon of molasses to a cup of warm water

2.Massage mixture into the hair.

(Make sure to completely cover the roots to stimulate hair growth)

3.After half an hour, rinse off with warm water. Then shampoo and condition as usual.

Tip 40: Rooibos tea has independent lab data to show it improves hair growth and condition hair. Brew and steep your Rooibos tea until cooled, then pour over hair as a hair rinse. Rinsing with Rooibos after showering also helps lessen frizz.

Tip 41: Make time to sleep and get enough shut-eye every night. You can indulge your strands whilst you sleep with a night time masque or leave-in conditioner.

Tip 42: Oil and loose braid your hair before going to bed to limit damage from when you are asleep. Silk pillowcases cause less friction when you move around at night and can help to prevent split ends whilst locking in your hair's natural oils.

Tip 43: If you want your hair to grow it is very important for you to manage your stress in positive ways. This means taking care of your health through diet and exercise and finding ways to relieve and avoid stress.

Tip 44: Wear your hair up so as to avoid hair snagging and to protect it from the elements. Be inventive and find new and exciting ways to wear your hair. Try to wear your hair out on special occasions only.

Tip 45: Chemicals from lice treatments can dry out hair and are absorbed into the blood stream. If you decide to continue using over the counter medicated headlice treatments, apply coconut or olive oil to your ends so they don't dry out.

Idea 14: **Natural Nit Treatment Recipe**

1.Add 20 - 30 ml of Neem oil to your shampoo

2.Leave in your hair for 10 minutes.

3.Rinse well and condition, before rinsing again.

Regular washing with Neem shampoo will help you get rid of nits for good.

Tip 46: Fine tooth combs for lice removal can damage your hair, therefore apply a generous amount of coconut oil to your hair to assist the comb in gliding through your hair and to suffocate nits.

Tip 47: Antifungal cremes that contain Miconazole Nitrate can reduce the growth of scalp fungus and improve circulation to the scalp. Applying these cremes to the roots of your hair 2-3times a week can improve the growth rate of your hair.

Warning: Pregnant and Breastfeeding mothers should see their health provider before use.

Tip 48: Herbs can be taken orally or used as a rinse to stimulate the scalp and hair follicles. Finding the right herbal mix can effectively condition and strengthen your hair. You can boil them into a tea and infuse them into an after showering hair rinse. Otherwise use a little essential oil mixed with your favourite oil and massage into the scalp.

Tip 49: Horsetail can be brewed into a tea and taken internally or applied as an after shower hair rinse. Its high silica content helps build protein, making hair stronger.

Tip 50: Traditional medicines have been used for hundreds of years to treat dandruff, increasing blood circulation, scalp cleansing and reducing inflammation. A combination of one or more Ayurvedic and Chinese Herbs may just be the missing link in helping you achieve longer healthier hair.

Tip 51: Scalp massages stimulate circulation to nourish hair follicles. After showering, massage the scalp vigorously with your favourite oil until it starts to feel warm or for at least 5minutes every day.

Idea 15: **Controlled Pulling 'How to'**

Controlled Pulling should never hurt or uproot any hairs, if it does you are pulling too hard

1.Start by placing your fingers on the scalp and moving the scalp back and forth like you are adjusting a wig

2.Grasp random chunks of hair firmly by the roots and tug gently

(Avoid asking another person to help you with this, as they are 99.5% likely to get carried away doing it at your expense!)

3.Continue this routine until you have "pulled" the hair all over your scalp.

Tip 52: Inverting your head helps get circulation to your scalp, you can try inversion whilst you massage with your favourite oils, when washing your roots and when combing your hair.

Idea 16: **How to Invert your hair whilst standing**

1.Bend at the waist

2.Hang your head forward and tuck your chin under so it touches your chest

3.Allow your hair to fall over the head so it hangs freely

Tip 53: See your Health practitioner and have your hormone levels checked. Also, if applicable, check the hormone levels on any birth control you may be taking.

Tip 54: It will take around three months for you to see changes in your hair when you adopt some of or all of these Tips and Ideas. Remember, patience is key to growing longer hair.

APPENDIX - (Cheat sheet) – Stuff you can try, buy, do and avoid

Stuff you can buy and try

Coconut oil

Oils – jojoba, avocado, mineral, almond & olive oil

Argan oil

Castor Oil

Henna – indigo, hendigo, cassia

Natural hair lighteners - cinnamon, honey or lemon

Miconazole nitrate crème

Coconut oil shampoo

Baking soda shampoo

Wide tooth wood comb

Silk or satin pillowcase

Apple cider vinegar rinses

Molasses hair masque

Banana hair masque

Showerhead filter

Swim cap

Soda water rinses

Trial shampooing variations

Deep conditioning shea butter hair masque

Rooibos tea rinses

Neem lice treatments

Aromatherapy essential oils

Ayurvedic herbal teas & rinses

Chinese medicine

Stuff you can eat and drink

Healthy food

Vitamin & mineral supplements

Apple cider vinegar

Clean water

Rooibos tea

Horsetail tea

Nuts

Bananas

Pumpkin seeds

Increase protein intake

Iron rich food

Ayurvedic herbs

Stuff you can do NOW

Scalp massages

Microtrims

Cold water rinses

Braiding hair at night

Wear loose hairstyles

Wearing hair up during the day

Gentle brushing

Don't fight genetics, embrace your curls and kinks

Sunshine

Inversion

Patience

Sock buns

Hair wrapping

Indian hair pulling

Beauty sleep

Protect ends during nit treatments

Lifestyle changes

Hormones checked

Protein treatments

Finger combing

Natural styling products

Varying the position of hair parting

Blood tests for nutritional deficiencies

Speak up when in the hairdresser's chair

Stuff you can avoid doing

Chemical hair dyes

Chemical hair treatments – perms & straightening

Using excessive heat - blow driers, straighteners, curling wands & scalding hot showers

Over zealous dry brushing/wet brushing

Avoiding stress

Excessive hair cuts

Rough use of plastic brushes and combs

Bleaching

Salt water, treated water and hard water

Too much Sun exposure

Alcohol based synthetic styling products

Repetitive hairstyling

Backcombing & hair teasing

Harsh shampoos

Overtight braids and ponytails

Yoyo and Crash dieting

The Last Word

If you'd like to read more about the *why* behind each of these tips and ideas please 'like' us on our Facebook page and we'll give you the 'heads up' on upcoming specials and promotions for the original book *'The Lush Long Hair Care Guide'*.

Connect with Me Online:

Twitter: www.twitter.com/Cousinlt

Facebook: www.facebook.com/LushLongHairCareGuide

Website www.thelushlonghaircareguide.com

Made in the USA
San Bernardino, CA
08 July 2013